TABLE OF CONTENTS

INTRODUCTION

Get Control of Your Blood Sugar is designed to rescue you from the wild ups and downs of the blood sugar roller coaster. Whether you have type 2 diabetes, prediabetes, or a high risk of developing the disease, reining in wildly fluctuating blood sugar levels can: slow, stop, or even reverse the condition; tame your current symptoms and help warm off long-term complications; and lessen, delay, or prevent the need for a lifetime of pills and shots.

In the opening chapters, you'll learn about the immediate and longer-term benefits of blood sugar control. In chapter 3, you'll learn about individual blood sugar readings, ideal blood sugar ranges, HbA1c measurements, and how to set blood sugar goals that reflect a level of control appropriate for you. Chapter 4 covers the practical aspects of testing your blood sugar, from selecting testing supplies and setting up a testing schedule to making sense of the results. In chapter 5, you'll learn about the lifestyle tools you can use to control blood sugar. Finally, we'll look at medication options in chapter 6.

CHAPTER 1
Immediate Benefits of Control

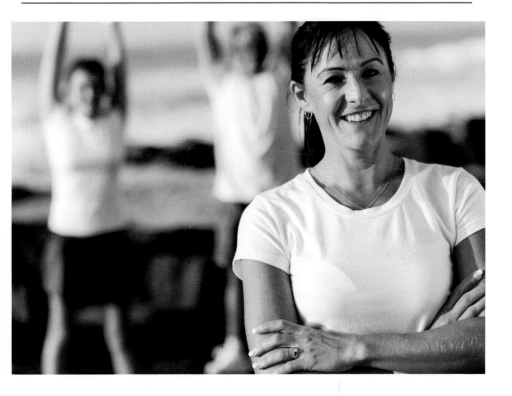

Understanding the immediate improvements you'll experience can provide powerful motivation to start reining in your runaway blood sugar. In the following pages, we discuss some of the concrete ways in which you will be rewarded right away for getting your blood sugar levels under control, including:

- Increased energy
- More restful sleep
- Decreased appetite
- Improved physical performance
- Heightened brain power
- More stable moods and emotions
- Fewer sick days

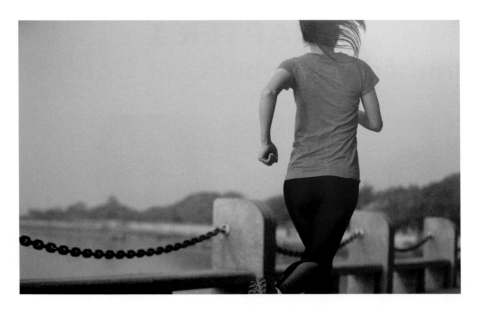

Increased Energy

Elevated blood sugar reduces your overall energy level. Remember, high blood sugar is a sign that not enough sugar is getting into your body's cells, where it is used for energy. The fuel is there; it's just stuck in the bloodstream, kind of like a fleet of gasoline trucks that drive around aimlessly instead of unloading at your local gas station. This shortage of fuel inside the body's cells causes sleepiness and sluggishness. Even if the blood sugar is only elevated temporarily, the lack of energy will be noticeable during that time. As soon as the blood sugar returns to normal, the energy level usually improves. So forget the gimmicky "energy drinks." If you want more energy, control your diabetes!

More Restful Sleep

We all know how important a good night's sleep is to feeling well and being productive the following day. Unfortunately, diabetes makes you more prone to developing sleep disorders, including sleep apnea, a potentially life-threatening disorder in which the sleeper snores loudly and actually stops breathing multiple times throughout the night. Poor blood sugar control also reduces the *quality* of your sleep. If you've ever woken up from a really long night's sleep feeling as though you hardly got any rest at all, it may

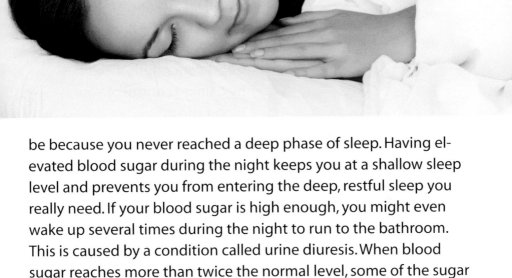

be because you never reached a deep phase of sleep. Having elevated blood sugar during the night keeps you at a shallow sleep level and prevents you from entering the deep, restful sleep you really need. If your blood sugar is high enough, you might even wake up several times during the night to run to the bathroom. This is caused by a condition called urine diuresis. When blood sugar reaches more than twice the normal level, some of the sugar spills into the urine, dragging a lot of water along with it. As the bladder fills, it wakes you up. The result may be frequent nighttime urination and even bedwetting. If the thought of a restful, uninterrupted, "dry" night's sleep appeals to you, start getting your blood sugar levels under control now!

Decreased Appetite

It might sound totally backward, but high blood sugar levels tend to make you crave more food—especially carbohydrate-rich food. Remember, when it comes to appetite, it's not the amount of sugar in the bloodstream that counts; it's how much of that sugar gets into the body's cells. If not enough is getting into the cells, particularly the cells that regulate appetite, the body is going to feel hungry no matter how much food is eaten. Given that weight control is so important to both diabetes management and to your long-term health, it makes all the sense in the world to control your diabetes as best you can.

Improved Physical Performance

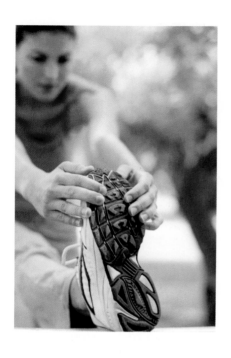

Elevated blood sugar can reduce your strength, flexibility, speed, and stamina. So whether you're an aspiring athlete or just hoping to make it up a flight of stairs, you can immediately boost your physical abilities by gaining control of your blood sugar.

Muscles prefer sugar as fuel when they make quick, intense movements. When the sugar in the bloodstream can't get into the muscle cells, therefore, strength suffers. Extra sugar in the bloodstream also leads to something called glycosylation of connective tissues, in which sugar coats tendons and ligaments, limiting their ability to stretch properly. Muscle stiffness, strains, and pulls are common in people with high blood sugar levels. High blood sugar also gunks up the connections between muscles and nerves, resulting in dulled reflexes and slower reaction times. And extra sugar in the bloodstream limits the ability of red blood cells to pick up oxygen in the lungs and transport it to working muscles, causing rapid fatigue and restricted cardiovascular/aerobic capacity. So if you want to be able to perform well physically—during sports, exercise, or simple everyday activities—control your diabetes!

Heightened Brain Power

Blood sugar levels influence more than your muscles, ligaments, and tendons, however. They affect your brain, too. High blood sugar limits your ability to focus, remember, perform complex tasks, and be creative. Studies have repeatedly and consistently shown that mental performance suffers during periods of high blood sugar. As blood sugar goes up, so do mental errors and the time it takes to perform basic tasks. Wide variations in blood sugar levels, from early-morning lows to post-meal spikes, have also been shown to hinder intellectual function. If you have noticed a decline in your mental abilities, tightening control of your diabetes might be the answer. Likewise, if you want to perform as well as you possibly can, be vigilant about tracking and balancing those blood sugar levels.

More Stable Moods and Emotions

Besides intellectual performance, your brain is also responsible for maintaining your emotional balance. The fact is, your moods change along with your blood sugar level. Achieving normal blood sugar levels and keeping them there can go a long way toward improving your mood and your emotional stability. That's not to say that you will become an instant optimist or the life of the party. But the way you interact with your family, friends, coworkers, and even perfect strangers truly can impact your success and happiness in life. If you want to be on a more even keel, try evening out your blood sugar levels.

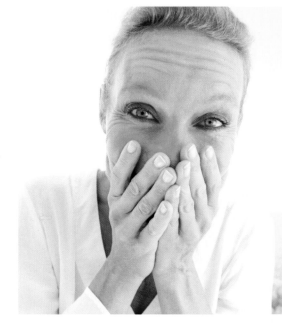

Fewer Sick Days

Bacteria and viruses love sugar. They gobble it up and use it to grow and multiply. When blood sugar levels are up, the levels of sugar in virtually all of the body's tissues and fluids rise as well. That makes the diabetic body an ideal breeding ground for infection. If you ignore your high blood sugar levels, therefore, you are essentially supplying extra nutrients to the bad guys. Think of it as aiding and abetting the enemy. Everything from common colds and the flu to sinus infections and vaginal yeast infections are more common when blood sugar levels are elevated. And once illnesses and infections set in, they are much more difficult to shake when blood sugar is high. In fact, people with diabetes are much more likely to die from pneumonia or influenza than are people who do not have diabetes. Research has shown that people who have better blood sugar control spend significantly fewer days absent from work, sick in bed, and restricted from their usual activities. So if you don't like—or can't afford—to get sick, take better care of your diabetes!

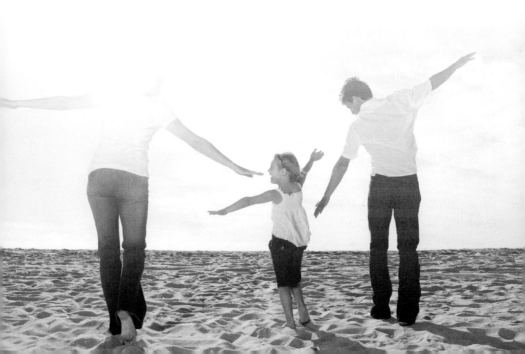

CHAPTER 2
Control's Preventive Power

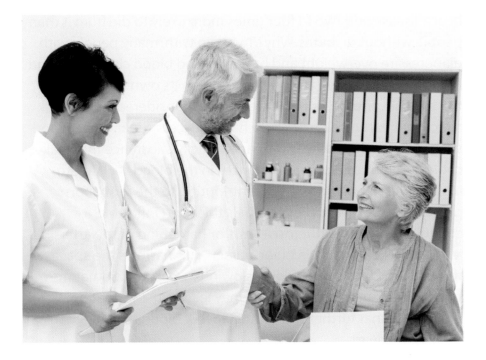

There may be no better motivation for stabilizing your blood sugar than the fear of living with—or dying from—the devastating long-term complications that are likely to occur if you don't. So in this chapter, we'll look at the proven long-term benefits of quality blood sugar management, including:

- Improved heart health
- Better blood flow
- Healthy kidneys
- Proper nerve function
- Less nerve pain
- Clear vision
- Mental soundness
- Healthy teeth and gums
- A positive outlook

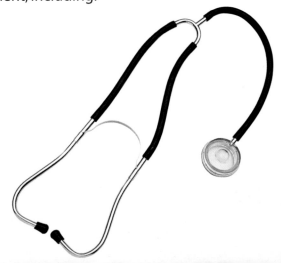

Improved Heart Health

Despite the long list of health problems diabetes can cause, heart disease is what ultimately kills the majority of people with diabetes. People with diabetes are at least twice as likely to develop heart disease and two to four times more likely to die from it than people without diabetes. Why? To begin with, many people with diabetes are overweight and have elevated blood cholesterol and blood pressure levels, any one of which on its own increases the risk of heart disease. But diabetes itself is considered a major risk factor for heart disease because having excess sugar in the bloodstream threatens the heart. Sugar is a sticky substance that makes cholesterol, fat, and other substances in the blood stick to the interior walls of blood vessels, contributing to the formation of plaque. Plaque makes blood vessels thick and inflexible, a condition known as atherosclerosis, or hardening of the arteries. The thickening of the blood vessel walls narrows the space through which the blood flows, slowing its passage. Sometimes pieces of plaque break off, which may lead to the formation of blood clots that further restrict the flow of blood to vital organs such as the heart.

The good news: Improving blood sugar control dramatically reduces the risk of heart disease. In addition to preventing the formation of much of the plaque that clogs blood vessels, better diabetes management also frequently leads to reductions in blood cholesterol and blood pressure levels. Plus, the positive lifestyle steps you take to control blood sugar further reduce your risk of heart disease.

Better Blood Flow

In addition to the heart, a number of other vital body parts require large amounts of oxygen and depend on healthy blood vessels to deliver an unobstructed flow of oxygen-rich blood. The most important of these is the brain. When a blood vessel leading to the brain becomes clogged with sticky plaque, the brain cells normally fed by that vessel do not receive enough oxygen and quickly die.

This is called a stroke. The risk of stroke is two to four times higher for people who have diabetes than for people who do not have it.

The muscles in the legs also depend on a reliable and substantial flow of blood. When blood vessels that feed the legs become clogged, the leg muscles don't get sufficient oxygen, which can lead to pain or cramping during exercising or walking. This condition is called claudication. Blood vessel disease in the legs is *20 times* more common in people with diabetes than in those without it. Claudication occurs in 15 percent of people who have had diabetes for 10 years and 45 percent of those who have had diabetes for 20 years.

The good news: Tightening blood sugar control, along with all the other changes and lifestyle improvements that come with it, will help blood flow more freely to all the vital body parts. For people with diabetes who have already developed circulatory problems, symptoms often decrease as blood sugar levels improve.

Healthy Kidneys

Visit any kidney dialysis center and check the charts of the people who sit there for hours a day, several days a week, with tubes in their arms, hooked up to machines that filter waste products, toxins, and other undesirable substances from their blood. Diabetic. Diabetic. Not diabetic. Diabetic. Diabetic. Get the idea?

Diabetes is the leading cause of kidney failure, accounting for 44 percent of new cases of kidney disease. More than 200,000 Americans with diabetes have received kidney transplants or are receiving dialysis treatment. Approximately 50,000 Americans with diabetes begin treatment for end-stage renal (kidney) disease each year. Minorities, especially African Americans and Hispanics, who have type 2 diabetes are highly susceptible to kidney disease, but everyone with elevated blood sugar levels is at risk. Elevated blood sugar damages the tiny blood vessels, called capillaries, which form and nourish the filters within the kidneys.

The good news: Tightening blood sugar control dramatically reduces the risk of kidney disease. In fact, major studies examining the effect of blood sugar levels on kidney disease found that every 30 mg/dl drop in average blood sugar leads to a 30 percent reduction in the risk of kidney disease.

Proper Nerve Function

The nervous system is like the body's electrical wiring, relaying signals that control voluntary and involuntary functions throughout the body. A portion of that interior wiring, called the autonomic nervous system, controls the body's involuntary activities—all of the basic, "behind the scenes" functions, such as the beating of the heart, the digestion of food, the regulation of body temperature, the maintenance of balance, and the physical response to sexual stimulation, that occur without conscious thought or direction on our part.

Nerves are like any other living tissue in the body: They burn sugar for energy, and they require an unobstructed blood supply to provide them with oxygen and other nutrients. Excess sugar in the blood appears to cause two main problems for the nervous system. First, it interferes with the blood supply to the nerves (as it does to other tissues and organs) by contributing to plaque buildup in the blood vessel walls. Second, it seems to alter energy metabolism (the burning of sugar to fuel cell functions) in such a way that the nerves swell and the coating on the outside of the nerve fibers fails to do its job of insulating and protecting the nerves. When the nerves that regulate basic body functions are damaged in this way by high blood sugar levels, the condition is called autonomic neuropathy.

Population-based studies have shown that 60 to 70 percent of people with diabetes have some form of mild to severe nerve damage. For example, nearly 50 percent of all men with diabetes develop impotency within a decade of diagnosis, due mainly to malfunction of the nerves that produce an erection. Women with diabetes are more likely than women without it to suffer from vaginal dryness, again as a result of damage to nerves that control sexual response. Nerve damage can also lead to delayed digestion, a condition known as gastroparesis that affects upwards of 30 percent of people with type 2 diabetes. Gastroparesis can cause painful bloating, and because it delays the peaking of blood sugar that normally occurs after a meal, it can make diabetes even harder to control. Postural hypotension, yet another condition caused by damage to nerves, is twice as common in people with diabetes. It's a type of low blood pressure that occurs upon sitting or standing and that can lead to dizziness and fainting.

The good news: Blood sugar control is an effective means for preventing all forms of autonomic neuropathy. And while autonomic neuropathy is not always reversible once it has developed, the condition may regress slightly or at least won't progress any further once blood sugar levels are returned to normal.

Less Nerve Pain

As previously mentioned, 60 to 70 percent of all people with diabetes develop some form of nerve damage in their lifetime. Of those, most develop a form called peripheral neuropathy—malfunction of the nerves serving the limbs, especially the lower legs and feet. In its early stages, peripheral neuropathy expresses itself as tingling or numbness. But as it progresses and nerves become inflamed, it can cause constant and sometimes severe pain. While there are several conventional and alternative medical treatments for painful neuropathy, many sufferers find little or no relief.

The good news: Tight blood sugar control can help to minimize the pain and slow the progression of peripheral neuropathy. Even better, if it is initiated early enough in the course of diabetes, tight control may actually prevent peripheral neuropathy from developing in the first place.

Clear Vision

In the back of the eye is a sensitive layer of tissue called the retina that acts much like the film in a camera. The retina receives and records light from the outside world. Those images in light are then converted into electrical signals that are transmitted to the brain to produce vision. A network of capillaries provides the living cells of the retina with oxygen and nutrients. Elevated blood sugar levels, however, weaken these tiny blood vessels. As a result, they may swell, leak, or grow in unhealthy ways, blocking light from ever reaching the retina. This condition is called diabetic retinopathy.

Diabetes is the leading cause of new cases of blindness among adults ages 20 to 74. Diabetic retinopathy accounts for 12,000 to 20,000 new cases of blindness each year. In fact, roughly one of every five people with type 2 diabetes already has retinopathy when they are diagnosed with diabetes. Glaucoma, cataracts, and diseases of the cornea (the transparent outer covering of the eyeball) are also more common in people with diabetes and contribute to the high rate of blindness among this population.

The good news: Tight blood sugar control reduces the risk of retinopathy. Every 30 mg/dl reduction in average blood sugar lowers the risk of retinopathy by approximately 30 percent. For those with existing retinopathy, tightening blood sugar control slows the progression significantly.

Mental Soundness

With aging comes increased risk for a number of health problems. Few instill as much fear as Alzheimer's disease, a progressive and ultimately fatal disease that destroys brain cells, causing increasingly severe problems with memory, thinking, and behavior. Today, it affects more than five million Americans and is the sixth-leading cause of death in the U.S. Currently, there is no cure for Alzheimer's. Damaged blood vessels in the brain are believed to play a role in the development of Alzheimer's. And recent research suggests that people with diabetes are more than twice as likely to develop Alzheimer's compared to those with normal glucose tolerance.

The good news: If you have type 2 diabetes, tight blood sugar control can reduce your risk of Alzheimer's disease to that of the general non-diabetic population.

Healthy Teeth and Gums

Adults with diabetes have two times the risk of developing gum disease (periodontitis) as do their peers without diabetes. Almost one-third of people with diabetes have severe gum disease. Specifically, those with type 2 diabetes have greater plaque buildup and more bacteria below the gumline; as a result, their gums bleed more easily, and they commonly experience loosening and loss of teeth. Once a gum infection starts, it can take a long time to eradicate it when blood sugar is out of whack. Conversely, research has shown that having periodontal disease may make it more difficult for people who have diabetes to control their blood sugar levels.

The good news: Good blood sugar control can help prevent dental problems. The lower the average blood sugar level, the lower the risk of gum disease and tooth loss.

Flexible Joints

Joint mobility problems, including conditions such as frozen shoulder, trigger finger, and clawing of the hand, affect approximately 20 percent of people with diabetes, and high blood sugar is the root cause. Excess sugar in the blood sticks to collagen, a protein found in bone, cartilage, and tendons. When collagen becomes sugar-coated, it thickens and stiffens, preventing joints from moving smoothly through their full range of motion and often causing joint pain.

The good news: Keeping your blood sugar levels near normal reduces your risk of developing joint mobility problems. If you already have limited range of motion in your shoulders, hands, fingers, or other joints, lowering blood sugar levels may help improve your range of motion and limit the pain associated with stiff joints.

A Positive Outlook

Blood sugar levels have a direct effect on our mental well-being. It is common for people with diabetes to feel down when their blood sugar levels are up. Depression is three to four times more common in adults with diabetes than in the general population. The mechanism of this increased risk is not entirely known. Since depression is often biochemical in nature, elevated sugar levels in the brain may play a direct role. It could also be related, at least in part, to the extra stress associated with living with a chronic illness. Certainly, developing complications from diabetes can instill a feeling of helplessness, a definite contributing factor in the onset of depression.

The good news: Improving your blood sugar levels can make you a happier person. Researchers at Harvard Medical School and the Joslin Diabetes Center studied the effects of blood sugar control on mood and disposition. They found that people with lower blood sugar levels reported a higher overall quality of life. Significantly better ratings were given in the areas of physical, emotional, and general health and vitality.

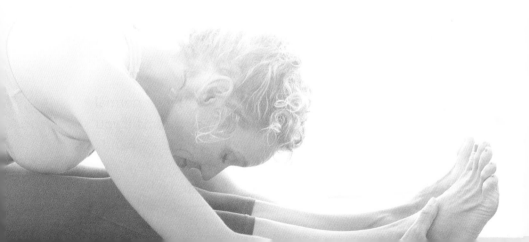

CHAPTER 3
Set Your Targets

To know where you stand right now and where you want to go in terms of blood sugar control, you need tools for measuring your progress and goals that will tell you when you've arrived.

Evaluating Your Control

Monitoring your blood sugar when you have diabetes or pre-diabetes is much like paying attention when you drive. You look ahead, behind, and to the sides so you can assess the conditions of the road and avoid other cars. You steal quick glances at the speedometer so you can maintain a safe speed and avoid costly tickets (and accidents). And you heed the warning lights on the dashboard so you'll know when it's time to take your vehicle in for fuel, maintenance, or repairs.

Ignoring your blood sugar levels, on the other hand, is like driving with a blindfold on. Sooner or later, you're going to crash.

To properly manage your diabetes, you'll have to make many important choices every day. To avoid "driving blind" as you make those choices, you need to be able to "see" where your blood sugar level is and how it's been behaving in response to your "course adjustments." To gain these essential insights, you need to test your blood sugar levels often and have HbA1c tests performed regularly. Of course, you also need to have an idea of where you want to end up—in other words, where your blood sugar levels should be to give yourself the best chance of avoiding devastating diabetes complications. And that means setting goals.

Individual Blood Sugar Readings

Individual blood sugar readings are essential for evaluating your blood sugar control (or lack thereof). These are the readings you get by pricking your finger (or an alternate site) and placing the resulting drop of blood on a test strip, which you then insert into a portable blood glucose meter. The meter then measures and reports your current blood sugar level.

Regularly gathering, recording, and reviewing your individual blood sugar "numbers" in this way serves several important purposes: **(1)** It provides a measuring stick for assessing your current state of blood sugar control. **(2)** It lets you track your progress from one point in time to another. **(3)** It reveals where improvements need to be made. **(4)** It teaches you the impact of your daily activities and choices. You can see, almost immediately, what works and what doesn't when it comes to keeping your blood sugar in a healthy range. Such prompt feedback not only provides you with a tool for tracking your control, it allows you to take action at once to bring a high or low level back into a healthier range.

Your blood sugar levels naturally vary throughout the day and from day to day, depending on a variety of factors, such as when you ate your last meal, exercised, and took any prescribed diabetes medication. By taking multiple readings each day and then averaging together all of the readings from the last one or two weeks, you can get additional insight into your level of control. Indeed, some glucose meters automatically calculate the average of your recent readings for you.

However, quality blood sugar control doesn't just mean having the lowest average. It also requires stability, because blood sugar readings that bounce from high to low aren't healthy, even when they result in an average that doesn't look so bad. Consider, for example, the following two people, Matt and John:

BLOOD SUGAR READINGS	AVERAGE
Matt: 113, 97, 120, 135, 144, 100, 177, 83, 111	120
John: 53, 204, 188, 67, 170, 68, 80, 202, 48	120

Both men have the same average blood sugar level. But look at the *variation* in John's readings: His blood sugar is high half the time and low half the time. Matt's blood sugar levels, on the other hand, are more stable and consistent, with no wild upward or downward spikes.

Too much variability in blood sugar levels can affect a person's quality of life. Having an episode of low blood sugar can be dangerous as well as uncomfortable, because it can cause symptoms such as dizziness, weakness, and rapid heartbeat; left untreated, it can quickly lead to blurred vision, confusion, loss of consciousness, and coma. Experiencing such risky lows on a regular basis is like living life on a tightrope. A high level of blood sugar, conversely, saps energy and mental focus, and frequent highs can become a real drag on the body and mind. There is also evidence that excessive variability in blood sugar levels can cause damage to blood

IDEAL BLOOD SUGAR RANGES

	Fasting (Wake-Up) Range	Pre-Meal Range	Post-Meal Range (1–2 hours after eating)
No risk of hypoglycemia*	70–100 mg/dl	70–120 mg/dl	<140 mg/dl
Low risk of hypoglycemia**	70–120 mg/dl	70–140 mg/dl	<160 mg/dl
High risk of hypoglycemia***	70–100 mg/dl	80–160 mg/dl	<180 mg/dl

mg/dl means milligrams per deciliter

* Includes those who are not taking insulin or medications that can cause hypoglycemia (glyburide, glipizide, meglitinides).

** Includes those taking insulin once daily or oral medications that can cause hypoglycemia (glyburide, glipizide, meglitinides).

*** Includes those taking multiple insulin injections daily and those unable to detect hypoglycemia.

vessels, even if the overall average is within the preferred range. The preferred, or ideal, range for your blood sugar level depends on your current diabetes treatment regimen and how likely it is to cause hypoglycemia, or low blood sugar. That ideal range also varies based on when you take a reading—your ideal range will be different after a night of fasting than it will be an hour or two after a meal, for example. You can use the table on page 21 to determine your ideal fasting, pre-meal, and post-meal ranges. Once you know them, you can assess the quality of your blood sugar control by considering how often your readings fall within the appropriate ranges.

It is not necessary for your blood sugar to be in your ideal range every time you check it. Every person who has been diagnosed with diabetes has moments of weakness when it comes to managing the disease. As a general rule, if at least 75 percent (three out of four) of your readings are in the proper range, you're doing a pretty good job of controlling your blood sugar. If more than 10 percent (one out of ten) of your readings are below your ideal range or if more than 25 percent (one out of four) are above it, you may need some additional self-management education or an adjustment to your medication regime.

If your current blood sugar readings are well above your ideal ranges, it's reasonable to set temporary targets that fall between the two. For example, if you are not at risk for hypoglycemia but have blood sugars that are consistently above 200, an initial goal might be to get your readings into the 100 to 180 range. Once you've brought your sugar levels down into that target range, you can then aim for your ideal range(s).

HbA1c Measurements

The second essential tool for gauging your blood sugar control is a test that measures glycohemoglobin A1c, often referred to as HbA1c or simply A1c. The result of this simple blood test, arranged through your doctor's office, reflects your average blood sugar level over the previous two to three months, giving you insight into your blood sugar control over a longer term.

Inside your red blood cells is a protein called hemoglobin that carries oxygen from your lungs to your body's tissues. Sugar in the blood has a tendency to glycate, or stick to, this protein, forming glycohemoglobin. Once the glucose attaches to the hemoglobin, it stays there as long as the red blood cell lives, typically two to three months. Your red blood cells don't all die at once; old ones are constantly dying, and new ones are constantly being created. So at any one time, your red blood cells are a mix of the very old, the middle aged, and the quite young.

In someone without diabetes, roughly 4 to 6 percent of their hemoglobin is coated with sugar. In the person with diabetes, whose blood sugar levels are higher, more sugar attaches to the hemoglobin molecules; usually anywhere from 6 to more than 20 percent of the hemoglobin is sugar-coated. The A1c test measures this percentage. (A1c refers to a type of glucose-coated hemoglobin that is especially suited for gauging long-term blood sugar levels.) And because some of the hemoglobin molecules in the blood are older and some newer, the A1c result provides a good estimate of how high the blood sugar has been over the past two to three months.

That's why you should ask your doctor to order an A1c test for you every three months until your sugar levels and A1c are stable and within your target ranges. Once you've reached those goals, it's usually sufficient to have the A1c test every six months, unless your doctor orders more frequent testing.

It's true that several companies sell at-home A1c test kits, but you're probably better off having a professional draw your blood and send it to a laboratory for testing. (Many doctors' offices and virtually all hospitals can do this for you.) Although the at-home kits are reasonably accurate, they require multiple steps. If any of the steps are not performed exactly right, the test will be useless and you'll have wasted your money on the cost of the kit.

When you use the results from the A1c and the individual blood sugar tests you perform yourself, you get a fuller and more accurate picture of your level of control. Using the individual results alone would be like trying to judge a baseball batter's ability by looking at a day or two of single at-bats. Just as a great hitter will make an out or have a bad day sometimes, a person with good control will have the occasional high or low. So to truly gauge the player's batting skill, you need to also see his season average. And to evaluate your level of sugar control, you need to know your A1c.

A1c	AVERAGE BLOOD SUGAR
5%	97
6%	126
7%	154
8%	183
9%	212
10%	240
11%	269
12%	298
13%	326
14%	355

To translate your A1c result into an average blood sugar level, use the table to the left, or this formula: $(A1c \times 28.7) - 46.7 = $ average blood sugar

There's another reason testing A1c is so important. Research has shown it is closely linked to the risk of developing diabetic complications. Essentially, the higher the A1c, the greater the risk of developing eye, kidney, nerve, and heart problems.

That is why you should try to keep your A1c as near to normal as possible. In most cases, that equates to an A1c of 6 to 7 percent. A looser A1c of 7 to 8 percent may be a more appropriate target for anyone in whom an episode of hypoglycemia would be especially dangerous, including:

• Anyone who is susceptible to low blood sugar but suffers from hypoglycemia unawareness, a condition in which the individual is unable to detect the warning symptoms of a dropping blood sugar level until it is too late for them to help themselves.

• Anyone who has significant heart disease, because the rapid heartbeat and overall physical stress placed on the body during an episode of hypoglycemia can be particularly dangerous for a person who has an already weakened heart.

• Anyone who works in an extremely high-risk profession (taxi driver, trucker, construction worker, etc.), where experiencing dizziness, blurred vision, confusion, or loss of consciousness due to hypoglycemia could be devastating.

• A young child who can't communicate hypoglycemia symptoms.

On the other hand, a tighter A1c target of 5 to 6 percent may be appropriate for women who are pregnant or preparing to become pregnant, individuals planning for surgery, and anyone looking to slow or reverse existing diabetes complications.

Keep in mind that achieving these A1c targets may take time, especially if your current A1c is very high. Since the test is usually done every three months, it is reasonable to aim for an A1c that's one or two percentage points lower at each test.

Your Specific Target Ranges

When you put it all together, your ideal aim is to have the lowest possible individual blood sugar and A1c levels without experiencing frequent or severe hypoglycemia. Occasional, mild episodes of low blood sugar are acceptable and not dangerous for most people with diabetes. But if low blood sugars become too frequent (occurring more than two or three times a week) or severe (causing seizures or loss of consciousness), you'll need to ease up on your targets. So before proceeding, you need to set your own specific targets, using the information just discussed. Be sure to discuss those targets with your diabetes care team. Set targets for:
• Blood sugar, fasting range (upon waking)
• Blood sugar, pre-meal range (right before eating)
• Blood sugar, post-meal range (1–2 hours after eating)
• Your Ac1 target

CHAPTER 4
Testing Your Blood Sugar

You've set your sights on controlling your blood sugar levels. You've even specified exactly where you want your blood sugar levels to be. Now it's time to see where you actually stand.

Testing Supplies

To perform the individual blood sugar monitoring that is so essential to good control, you need three main supplies: **(1)** a blood glucose meter, **(2)** the testing strips for that meter, and **(3)** a lancet or lancing device to draw the small amount of blood you'll need for testing. You will also need instruction in using the supplies you choose. Your doctor, certified diabetes educator, and/or pharmacist can give you a hands-on demonstration to ensure that you are using your equipment properly. Meter manufacturers also typically have hotlines that consumers can access in order to get answers and advice about their specific meters. Take advantage of these resources so that you can confidently and correctly measure your blood sugar levels as often as necessary for good control.

When it comes to choosing a meter, remember that quality diabetes management requires accurate and frequent blood sugar testing. Selecting a meter with the desirable qualities listed below should help make frequent testing less of a hassle.

- Fast (some meters take just seconds to produce a reading)

- Simple to use (fewer steps mean a quicker process and less chance for user error)

- Provides downloadable results (making it quick and easy to share your results with your diabetes care team)

- Requires very little blood (1 microliter or less is ideal)

• Easy to read (especially if you are visually impaired, choose a meter with a very large display or one that "talks")

The accuracy of just about every blood sugar meter on the market is pretty good. The values these meters produce typically fall within 15 percent of the reading a laboratory would produce on a blood sample taken at the same time. That's true, however, only if you use the correct testing technique.

With the advent of alternate-site testing—using meters that can test blood taken from places other than the sensitive fingertips, such as the forearm—blood sugar testing that's virtually pain free has become a reality. But be aware that alternate-site testing can be difficult with meters that require 1 microliter of blood or more. Also, a reading taken from the arm or leg may lag several minutes behind a reading taken from the fingertip. So if you suspect that your blood sugar is dropping quickly (after exercise or if you feel hypoglycemic) or rising quickly (after meals), blood taken from your fingertip will provide a more accurate reading than a sample taken from an alternate site.

To make it more likely that you will perform the frequent blood sugar testing that is so conducive to good control, you may find it helpful to have more than one meter. Having multiple identical meters makes testing more convenient (you can keep one in the kitchen and one in the bedroom, for example, or one at work and one at home) and ensures that if one of your meters isn't functioning or gets misplaced, you will have an equivalent backup available. Some meter companies will even send you an extra meter at no charge in an effort to win your loyalty and keep you purchasing their test strips.

When choosing a device for drawing your blood, you'll also want to opt for features and methods that will encourage—or at least won't discourage—frequent testing. For example:

COMMON TESTING PROBLEMS

ISSUE	SPECIFICS	SOLUTION
Insufficient blood	If not enough blood is applied to the test area on the strip, the reading may be artificially low.	Dose the strip adequately, as the meter manufacturer instructs. If you suspect a strip contained too little blood, ignore the result and start over with a new strip.
Improper coding	For most meters, you must enter a code number or chip/strip for each new vial or box of strips. If the meter is not coded for that specific package of strips, the readings may be inaccurate.	Every time you begin a new box or vial of strips, code your meter according to the manufacturer's instructions.
Outdated strips	Using test strips that are outdated may produce inaccurate readings.	Check the expiration date before buying and again before starting a vial or box of strips.
Heat or humidity	Heat and humidity will cause test strips to spoil and produce false readings.	Keep your strips sealed in their packaging and away from extreme temperatures. Do not leave test strips in your vehicle!
Dirt/impurities	Having substances like food or grease on your finger or other test site will impact the readings.	Ensure that your test site is clean when you check your blood sugar.

• Use the thinnest-gauge lancet you can find. (The higher the gauge, the thinner the lancet.) Thin lancets are less painful and cause less scarring than thicker lancets. Change the lancet at least once a day so the tip doesn't become dull.

• Use a lancing pen that allows you to adjust the depth of the stick, and turn it to the lightest possible setting that still produces a sufficient blood sample for your meter.

• For finger-stick testing, prick the side of your fingertip rather than the fleshy pad on the front. To obtain a sufficient blood drop after pricking, "milk" your finger by squeezing it, starting at the base and moving toward the tip.

• Opt for alternate-site testing (using your arm or leg, for example) whenever appropriate. It is almost always less painful than sticking your finger, and the readings taken at alternate sites are accurate as long as your blood sugar is not rising or dropping quickly at the time of the blood draw.

Before you go out and buy a meter at a local pharmacy, ask your doctor or diabetes educator if any free samples are available. Most meter manufacturers provide free sample meters for distribution to patients, in the hope that more patients will choose their meters and purchase their test strips for years to come. Most health insurance programs, including Medicare, Medicaid, and private insurance, cover the costs of meters, test strips, and lancets. You might want to consider using a reputable mail-order pharmacy or diabetes supply service; such operations will typically coordinate the insurance paperwork and ship your supplies directly to you as needed.

Deciding How Often to Test

What follows are some testing recommendations that vary based on whether you have been diagnosed with type 2 diabetes or prediabetes as well as on which, if any, diabetes medication you currently use. Find the schedule that applies to your current situation, and review the schedule with your diabetes care team before proceeding.

For those with prediabetes or those at high risk who take no diabetes medications: This testing schedule is for those diagnosed with prediabetes or with a high risk of developing diabetes who do not use any oral or injectable medications or insulin for their condition. Each week, you should test your blood sugar four times: just before breakfast one day, just before lunch another day, just before dinner on a third day, and at bedtime on a fourth day. The following is an example of how you might set up this schedule:

Sunday: no testing required
Monday: before breakfast
Tuesday: no testing required
Wednesday: before lunch
Thursday: no testing required
Friday: before dinner
Saturday: at bedtime

This schedule of testing will help you and your diabetes care team determine if your blood sugar remains in a healthy range throughout the day.

For those with type 2 diabetes who don't take insulin: This testing schedule is for those who have been diagnosed with type 2 diabetes but who do not take any insulin for their condition. This schedule applies whether or not any oral medication or any injectable incretin (exenatide, liraglutide, or pramlintide) is also being used.

Test your blood sugar every other day as follows: just before breakfast and then one to two hours after breakfast on day one, just before lunch and then one to two hours after lunch on day three, just before dinner and then one to two hours after dinner on day five, just before breakfast and one to two hours after breakfast on day seven, and so on. The following is an example of how you might set up this schedule:

Monday: before and 1–2 hours after breakfast
Tuesday: no testing required

Wednesday: before and 1–2 hours after lunch
Thursday: no testing required
Friday: before and 1–2 hours after dinner
Saturday: no testing required
Sunday: before and 1–2 hours after breakfast
Monday: no testing required

This testing schedule will allow you and your diabetes care team to see if your blood sugar remains normal before and after each of your meals. The wake-up and other pre-meal readings indicate whether your body is able to make enough of its own basal insulin (the baseline amount of insulin needed to offset the sugar that's naturally released by the liver between meals to maintain basic bodily functions). The after-meal readings indicate whether your pancreas can make enough bolus insulin (the additional burst of insulin needed at mealtimes to offset the carbohydrates from a meal).

For those with type 2 diabetes who take long-acting but not rapid-acting insulin: This testing schedule is for those who have been diagnosed with type 2 diabetes who are currently taking long-acting insulin (glargine, detemir, or NPH) but no rapid-acting (lispro, aspart, or glulisine) or premixed (50/50, 70/30, or 75/25) insulin. This schedule applies whether or not any oral medication or injectable incretin (exenatide, liraglutide, or pramlintide) is also being used.

Test your blood sugar at least twice a day, six days a week, as follows: On the first day, test just before and one to two hours after breakfast; on the second day, test just before and one to two hours after lunch; on the third day, test just before and one to two hours after dinner, and also at bedtime if it follows dinner by more than three hours; and on days four through six, repeat the schedule from days one through three. Take a break from testing on the last day of each week. The following is an example of how you might set up this schedule:

Monday: before and 1–2 hours after breakfast
Tuesday: before and 1–2 hours after lunch
Wednesday: before and 1–2 hours after dinner and at bedtime (if it's more than 3 hours after dinner)
Thursday: before and 1–2 hours after breakfast
Friday: before and 1–2 hours after lunch
Saturday: before and 1–2 hours after dinner and at bedtime (if it's more than 3 hours after dinner)
Sunday: no testing required

This testing schedule will allow you and your diabetes care team to see if your blood sugar remains normal before and after each of your meals.

For those with type 2 diabetes who take premixed insulin twice a day: This testing schedule is for those diagnosed with type 2 diabetes who currently inject premixed insulin (50/50, 70/30, or 75/25) twice each day rather than injecting long-acting (glargine, detemir, or NPH) and/or rapid-acting (lispro, aspart, or glulisine) insulin separately. This schedule applies whether or not any oral medication or injectable incretin (exenatide, liraglutide, or pramlintide) is also being used.

Each day of the week, test your blood sugar upon waking (before breakfast), at midday (before lunch), late in the afternoon (before dinner), and at bedtime. Also, as part of your weekly testing regimen, test your blood sugar one to two hours after breakfast on one day, one to two hours after lunch on another day, and one to two hours after dinner on a third day. The following is an example of how you might set up this schedule:

Sunday: before breakfast, before lunch, before dinner, and at bedtime
Monday: before breakfast, 1–2 hours after breakfast, before lunch, before dinner, and at bedtime
Tuesday: before breakfast, before lunch, before dinner, and at bedtime
Wednesday: before breakfast, before lunch, 1–2 hours after lunch, before dinner, and at bedtime
Thursday: before breakfast, before lunch, before dinner, and at bedtime
Friday: before breakfast, before lunch, before dinner, 1–2 hours after dinner, and at bedtime
Saturday: before breakfast, before lunch, before dinner, and at bedtime

The pre-meal checks are necessary because they allow you and your diabetes care team to evaluate the effectiveness of your insulin doses. The post-meal checks help to determine the optimal timing of your two daily injections.

For those with type 2 diabetes who take insulin at each meal:
This testing schedule is for those diagnosed with type 2 diabetes who currently inject rapid-acting insulin (lispro, aspart, or glulisine) at each meal and use long-acting insulin (glargine, detemir, or NPH) to cover their basal insulin needs. (No premixed insulin is used.) This schedule applies whether or not any oral medication or injectable incretin (exenatide, liraglutide, or pramlintide) is also being used.

Each day of the week, test your blood sugar just before every meal; just before your afternoon snack; just before your evening snack or, if you don't eat an evening snack, just before going to bed; prior to exercise; and before driving. Also, one day a week, test your blood sugar one to two hours after breakfast; on another day of the week, test one to two hours after lunch; and on a third day, test one to two hours after dinner. The following is a sample schedule:

Sunday: upon waking; before lunch; before your afternoon snack; before dinner; before your evening snack or at bedtime; and before exercising or driving

Monday: upon waking; 1–2 hours after breakfast; before lunch; before your afternoon snack; before dinner; before your evening snack or at bedtime; and before exercising or driving

Tuesday: upon waking; before lunch; before your afternoon snack; before dinner; before your evening snack or at bedtime; and before exercising or driving

Wednesday: upon waking; before lunch; 1–2 hours after lunch; before your afternoon snack; before dinner; before your evening snack or at bedtime; and before exercising or driving

Thursday: upon waking; before lunch; before your afternoon snack; before dinner; before your evening snack or at bedtime; and before exercising or driving

Friday: upon waking; before lunch; before your afternoon snack; before dinner; 1–2 hours after dinner; before your evening snack or at bedtime; and before exercising or driving

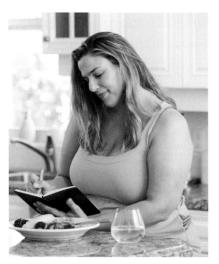

Saturday: upon waking; before lunch; before your afternoon snack; before dinner; before your evening snack or at bedtime; and before exercising or driving

The pre-meal tests are necessary because they allow you and your diabetes care team to evaluate the effectiveness of your insulin doses. The pre-driving and pre-exercise tests are for safety purposes. The post-meal tests help you and your team determine the optimal timing of your insulin doses.

Recording and Analyzing Your Results

To make your testing worthwhile, you need to review and learn from your results. By keeping organized and accurate records of your blood sugar tests and analyzing them on a regular basis, you can gain tremendous insight into your diabetes management program.

At its most basic, your record keeping system should include the date and time of every blood sugar test and the results you obtained from each one. As long as your blood sugar readings are consistently within your target ranges, it is not usually necessary to keep track of anything else. But if some of the readings are above or below target, it becomes necessary to figure out why. Was a high or low reading caused by the consumption of too much or too little food? The wrong type, dose, or timing of medication? An unusual amount of physical activity? Stress? Illness? Every time you use your records to make a sensible adjustment to your treatment regimen (whether in the type, amount, or timing of food, physical activity, or medication), your blood sugar control will get a little bit better.

If you need to figure out why your blood sugar levels are straying outside their target ranges, you will need to record other information in addition to your test results. The same is true if your treatment regimen calls for injecting insulin at mealtimes, an approach that requires you to account for meals and physical activity in determining the correct dose of insulin. In either situation, you will need to record the major factors that influence blood sugar levels, including:

• The type, dose, and timing of any diabetes medication (oral medication, noninsulin injection, and/or insulin)

• The grams of carbohydrate consumed in each meal and snack

• The type and length of exercise and other physical activities performed, such as housework, yard work, shopping, and extended walking

• Stresses that tend to affect blood sugar levels, such as physical illness, menstrual cycles, emotional events, and hypoglycemic episodes.

Learning how to interpret your self-monitoring records is also essential. Otherwise, your records are nothing more than pieces of paper covered with numbers. To get the most from your record keeping, it helps to organize the information so it will be easy to analyze. One way is to line up several days' data in columns so that you can detect blood sugar patterns that occur at particular times of day. If you notice that your blood sugar levels are consistently high or low at a certain point each day, it's easy to make the right kind of adjustment to bring it back in line.

ELLIE

	Before breakfast	After breakfast	Before lunch	After lunch	Before dinner	After dinner
Mon 3/3	95	166				
Wed 3/5			87	144		
Fri 3/7					77	158
Sun 3/9	99	190				
Tue 3/11			80	133		
Thu 3/13					100	202
Sat 3/15	81	175				

To see how this works, consider the table showing two weeks of blood sugar test results for Ellie. Ellie has type 2 diabetes and is currently taking no insulin or other medication for her diabetes. Her target blood sugar ranges are:

Fasting (before breakfast): 70–100
Before other meals: 70–120
After meals: <140

Notice how Ellie's pre-meal blood sugars are consistently near normal, but her after-meal readings are generally above her target range. It looks as though Ellie needs to work on managing her post-meal blood sugar, possibly through reduced carb intake at meals, some physical activity after meals, or the addition of a meal-time medication.

Now consider the results shown on the table for Debby. Debby is taking long-acting insulin once a day and oral diabetes medication at each meal. Her target blood sugar ranges are:

Fasting (before breakfast): 70–120
Before other meals: 70–140
After meals: <160

DEBBY

	Before breakfast	After breakfast	Before lunch	After lunch	Before dinner	After dinner	Bedtime
Mon 3/3	188	131					
Tue 3/4			102	122			
Wed 3/5					87	128	104
Thu 3/6	211	135					
Fri 3/7			110	114			
Sat 3/8					85	99	98

Debby's pre- and post-meal blood sugars are all pretty close to her targets, except for her level first thing in the morning. Debby's dose of long-acting insulin likely needs to be increased, or she needs to reduce her late-night snacking.

When you first begin testing, recording, and analyzing your own blood sugar levels, you should review your readings every couple of weeks. If they are fairly stable and within their target ranges, then monthly record reviews should be enough. But if you detect a pattern of readings that are out of range, bring them to the attention of your diabetes care team. Working with your team, you should be able to develop an effective solution for any control problem. And as your experience grows, there will likely come a time when you will be able to determine for yourself what minor adjustments to make in your treatment regimen to bring any errant levels back where they belong. (Even then, you'll need regular check-ins with your diabetes care team.)

Continuous Glucose Monitoring

Another tool in diabetes management technology is continuous glucose monitoring (CGM). Several systems are now available (by prescription) that provide blood sugar readings once every one to five minutes and emit warnings when the sugar level is heading for a high or low. These systems use a sensor, a thin metallic filament inserted just below the skin, to detect sugar in the fluid between fat cells. They come with a spring-loaded device that makes inserting the sensor quick and relatively painless. The information from the sensor is transmitted via radio signals to a receiver that looks like a cell phone. The receiver displays charts, graphs, and an estimate of the current blood sugar level. The transmitter and receiver are reusable, although the sensor filament must be replaced every few days or so, depending on the specific system and the body's ability to tolerate the filament.

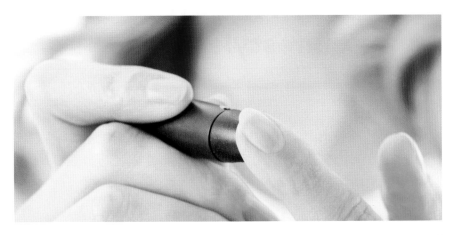

CGM devices are generally accurate to within about 15 percent of most finger-stick readings. They generate line graphs that depict sugar levels over the past several hours, allowing the user to detect trends and predict where blood sugar is headed. They use either vibration or a beeping noise to alert the wearer to impending high and low blood sugar levels. And computer or internet-based programs allow for detailed analysis of blood sugar levels over longer intervals of time.

Comparing finger-stick blood sugar testing to CGM is like comparing a photograph to a movie. CGM shows change and movement. It illustrates how virtually everything in daily life influences blood sugar levels. Used just once or twice, CGM can offer insight into the effectiveness of an individual's current diabetes management program. Worn on an ongoing basis, CGM makes it easier to keep blood sugars in range on a consistent basis with less risk of experiencing dangerous highs or lows.

CGM does have its drawbacks. It can be costly, and many health insurance plans resist covering it for people with type 2 diabetes. A CGM system requires some maintenance and technical know-how, and it's not always the most accurate testing method. It also still requires the user to enter the results from periodic finger-stick readings for calibration purposes, and improperly calibrating the device can lead to erroneous readings.

CHAPTER 5
Lifestyle Tools

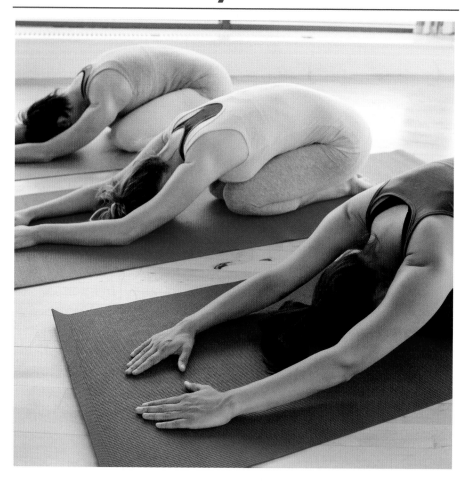

When you think of tight blood sugar control, you may assume it relies on medications. Surprise! Three lifestyle tools are essential for successfully managing your diabetes and blood sugar—healthy eating, physical activity, and stress management. Unleashing these lifestyle tools can make living in control far easier and can make life itself more enjoyable.

EATING FOR CONTROL

Understanding how your food choices affect your blood sugar is absolutely essential. No approach to tight control would be complete without a sound eating plan. There are three main factors you need to consider when making food choices:

1. Carbohydrates, because they have the greatest immediate impact on your blood sugar level;

2. Glycemic index, because in many cases the rate at which you digest is just as important as what you digest;

3. Calories, because you need to balance your energy intake against your energy expenditure.

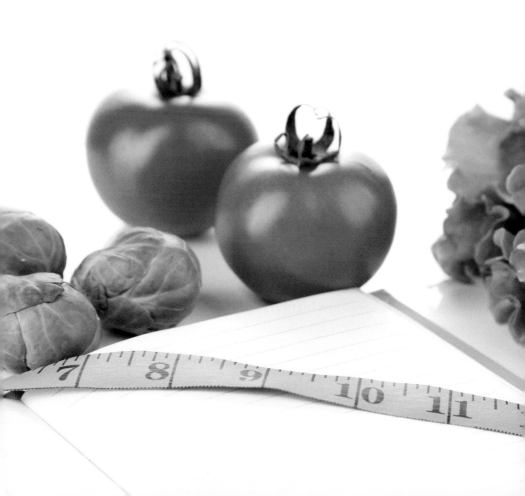

Controlling Carbohydrates

Carbohydrates include simple sugars such as sucrose (table sugar), fructose (fruit sugar), lactose (milk sugar), and corn syrup, as well as complex carbs, better known as starches. You can think of a simple sugar as an individual railroad car and a starch as a bunch of cars hooked together to make a train. Most starches are composed of many sugar molecules linked together.

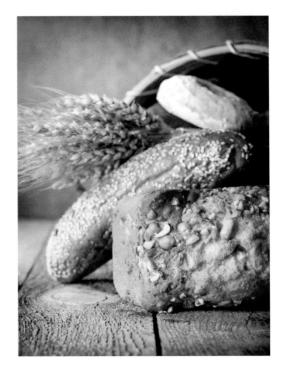

The carbs you eat are converted by your body into glucose, the sugar that circulates through your bloodstream to nourish your body's cells. Blood sugar is your body's primary fuel. To get the sugar out of your bloodstream and into your body's cells, your pancreas produces insulin. Consuming large amounts of carbohydrate places a heavy workload on the pancreas; so does eating carbs that digest very quickly, because the pancreas must pump out insulin at a furious rate to keep up with the sudden rush of sugar into the bloodstream. In people who are insulin resistant or who have a pancreas that has a hard time keeping up, there simply may not be enough insulin produced to keep the blood sugar level from going too high. Because carbs contain four calories per gram, consuming excessive amounts of carbohydrate will also contribute to weight gain, which exacerbates insulin resistance.

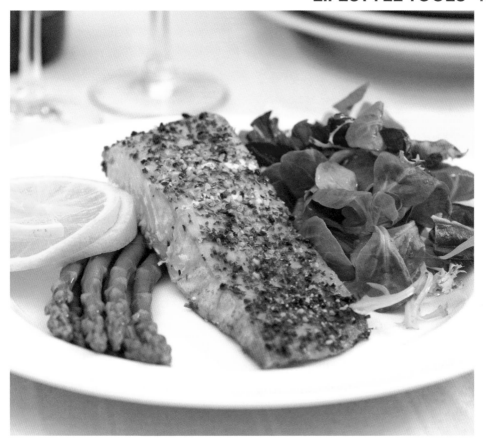

Carb Exchanging

Carb exchanging involves converting food types into grams of carbohydrate. It's based on the diabetic "exchange" system. Foods are grouped by categories, such as starches, vegetables, fruits, meats, and so on, with predetermined portion sizes. All food exchanges within a category have roughly equivalent nutritional value and impact on blood sugar levels. For example, one slice of bread counts as one "starch" exchange. It contains about 15 grams carbohydrate, 3 grams protein, and 80 calories. The same can be said of a half cup of cooked pasta, six saltine crackers, a third cup baked beans, or three cups of popcorn. In other words, three cups of popcorn can be "exchanged" for one slice of bread because it contains about the same carb, protein, and calorie count. (You'll find a detailed exchange list at the back of this book.)

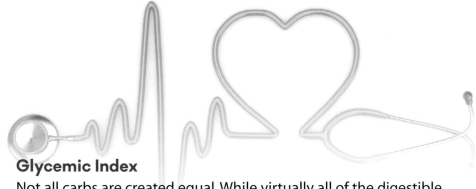

Glycemic Index

Not all carbs are created equal. While virtually all of the digestible carbs you consume will eventually be converted into blood glucose, some make the transition much faster than others. The rate at which different carbs are converted into blood glucose can be compared using something called the Glycemic Index (GI). The GI ranks foods on a scale from 0 to 100. At the top, with a score of 100, is pure glucose. Other foods are ranked in comparison to the absorption rate of pure glucose. (There's a list of GI scores for many common foods at the back of this book.)

What the score actually represents is the percentage of a food's carbohydrate content that turns into blood glucose within the two hours after the food is eaten.

Foods with a high GI score (70 or greater) tend to be digested and converted into glucose the fastest, producing a significant peak in blood sugar 30 to 45 minutes after they are eaten. Foods with a moderate GI score (56 to 69) digest a bit slower, resulting in a less pronounced peak in blood sugar approximately one to two hours after they are eaten. Foods with a low GI score (55 or less) have a slow, gradual effect on the blood sugar level: The peak is usually quite modest and may take several hours to occur.

Why care about GI scores? Because the effect that different foods have on your blood sugar is what really matters. In general, consuming primarily low-GI foods tends to make blood sugar easier to control. A diet of slowly digesting (low-GI) foods eases the workload on the pancreas, prevents post-meal spikes in blood sugar, and provides a satisfying form of slow-burning fuel.

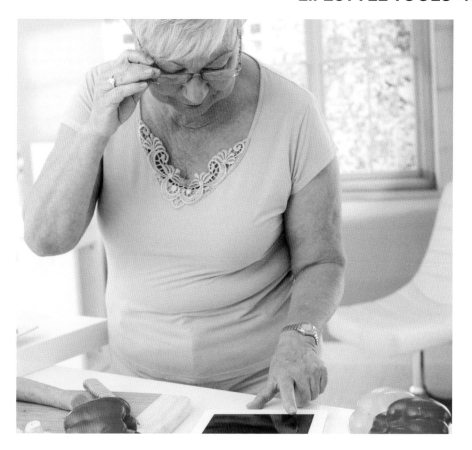

Calories and Weight Loss

The reason people with diabetes must pay such careful attention to calorie intake is that body fat interferes with insulin's action, causing or exacerbating insulin resistance. Each person's daily calorie needs are unique and are based on factors such as height, current weight, ideal weight, metabolism, and physical activity level. It's best to seek the guidance of a registered dietitian to help you figure out how many calories you should consume each day.

To lose excess body fat, you must burn more calories than you take in. Increasing your physical activity will help to create a calorie deficit. But exercise alone, with no change in caloric intake, rarely results in significant, sustainable weight loss. Most often, a combination of increased calorie expenditure and a modestly reduced calorie intake leads to the greatest weight loss over the long-term.

Falling for Less Fat

Falling for less fat boils down to choosing more foods that have less total fat and substituting healthier fats for some of the saturated fats you usually eat. Here are some tips:

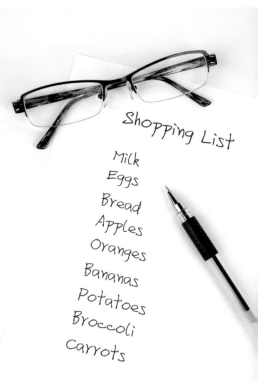

- Read food labels and opt more often for food with less total fat and less saturated fat.

- Eat a variety of fruits and vegetables, whole-grain products, beans, and nuts. Fruits and vegetables are naturally low in fat and provide loads of nutrients. Whole-grain foods and beans are low in fat but high in nutrients. Nuts, while not especially low in fat, are filled with mostly monounsaturated fats.

- Choose fish more often than poultry; choose poultry more often than red meat.

- Trim visible fat (it's saturated) from meat and fat and skin from poultry before eating.

- Instead of frying, try baking, broiling, roasting, or grilling.

- Use fat-free and low-fat milk products.

- Choose fats and oils that are trans fat free and have two grams or less of saturated fat per tablespoon.

THE TYPES OF FAT

There are three main types of fat: saturated, monounsaturated, and polyunsaturated. The more saturated a fat is, the more detrimental it can be when eaten to excess.

WHAT IT IS	WHAT IT DOES	WHERE IT'S FOUND
Saturated fats	These lead to more LDL molecules, the "bad" type of cholesterol.	Red meat, poultry, cheese, butter, full-fat dairy products; palm, coconut, and palm kernel oils.
Trans fats	Trans fats are created when unsaturated fats are "resaturated." This makes them act more like saturated fats in the body; they tend to raise total blood cholesterol. The use of trans fats is regulated in some cities and states.	Many breads, crackers, cookies, doughnuts, frozen pie crusts, deep-fried foods, fast foods, packaged and convenient foods.
Monounsaturated fats	These fats lower the number of LDL molecules.	Olive, canola, and peanut oils; olives; avocados; most nuts, including almonds, cashews, and pecans; peanuts and natural peanut butter.
Polyunsaturated fats	These can be divided into two types. *Omega 6 fatty acids* can cause water retention, raise blood pressure, increase blood clotting, and decrease "good" HDL cholesterol. *Omega 3 fatty acids* can lower blood cholesterol and heart disease risk by making blood less likely to clot.	Omega 6: Corn, sunflower, soybean, and cottonseed oils; many processed foods. Omega 3: Many fish, including wild salmon, mackerel, sardines, herring, anchovies, rainbow trout, bluefish, caviar, white albacore tuna; canola oil; flaxseed and flaxseed oil; walnuts and walnut oil; and dark green, leafy vegetables.

Opting for Less Salt

Too much sodium contributes to high blood pressure, which is especially common in and dangerous for people with type 2 diabetes. Decreasing your salt intake can help reduce your blood pressure, which cuts down on your risk of heart attack, stroke, and kidney problems. Here are some tips on reducing your sodium intake:

• Choose reduced-sodium or no-salt-added products.

• Buy fresh produce; there's no salt added.

• Use herbs, spices, lemon, lime, vinegar, or salt-free seasoning blends.

• Use fresh poultry, fish, and lean meats more often than canned, smoked, or processed types.

• Try low-sodium versions of soy sauce and teriyaki sauce.

• Take the saltshaker off the table. Always taste your food before adding any salt.

• Choose only small portions of foods that are pickled, cured, in broth, or bathed in soy sauce.

• When dining out, ask that your food be prepared without added salt, MSG, or high-sodium ingredients.

• Limit salty condiments such as ketchup, mustard, pickles, and mayonnaise.

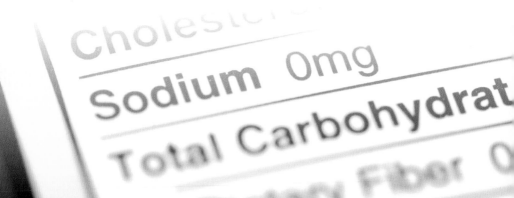

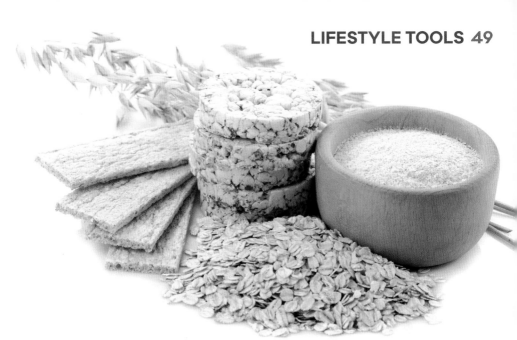

Fiber

Fiber has been proven effective in disease prevention, weight loss, and blood glucose control. It's naturally present in plants and therefore is a major nutritional component of fruits, vegetables, beans, nuts, seeds, and whole grains. Here are some tips on adding fiber to your diet:

- **Start out strong.** Choose a high-fiber hot cereal with fruit for breakfast.

- **Switch to whole grains.** Try brown rice, whole grain pastas and breads.

- **Eat the whole fruit.** The fiber is in the peel and the pulp. Foods with edible seeds, such as berries, are fiber filled, too.

- **Don't peel.** Paring off the skin of potatoes or other vegetables and fruits strips away fiber and nutrients, so leave it on. Corn and beans have edible skin, too.

- **Get big on beans.** Full of fiber, protein, B vitamins, and other nutrients, beans and lentils belong on any healthy menu. Eat beans or lentils three times a week.

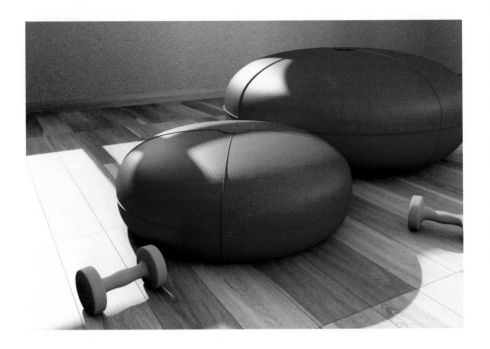

EXERCISING FOR GLUCOSE CONTROL

Exercise is another lifestyle tool essential to successfully managing your diabetes and blood sugar. Physical activity can take you where you want to go in terms of blood sugar control, weight loss, and a lower risk of diabetic complications. It can even prevent diabetes from developing in the first place.

Benefits of Being More Active
- Lower blood glucose
- Lower blood pressure
- Lower blood fats
- Better cardiovascular (heart and lung) fitness
- Weight loss and/or maintenance
- Improved sense of well-being

For more on fighting diabetes with exercise, see chapter 3 of the *You Can Reverse Diabetes* book in this set.

RELAXING FOR BETTER BLOOD SUGAR

When you feel stressed, your body naturally releases more sugar into your blood. It's the human condition, not the result of diabetes. But if you have diabetes and are trying to get control of your blood sugar, relieving stress should be part of your efforts.

Your Body Under Stress

Whether the cause of your stress is physical or emotional, your body will have a response. Stress causes an adrenaline rush, which increases the heart rate, dilates the pupils, tenses the muscles, causes sweating, stops digestion, and makes the liver release a jolt of sugar into the bloodstream for quick energy. In some scenarios, this stress response is helpful. However, we can have the same response to everyday mental stress, and that's less helpful. You don't want your blood pressure, heart rate, and blood sugar level to rise every time you're stuck in rush hour traffic.

The Stress Response and Diabetes

For people with diabetes, managing a stress response can be especially important. The stress hormones that cause the liver to secrete extra sugar into the blood in response to fear, anger, tension, or excitement also increase insulin resistance. For people without diabetes, the stress-induced rise in blood sugar is followed by an increase in insulin secretion, so the blood sugar spike is modest and momentary. For people with diabetes, however, stress can cause blood sugar to rise quickly and stay high for quite a while.

Reducing Stress

We all have some degree of stress in our lives. You can't cut out stress completely. However, you want to minimize its impact on your life. Start by figuring out what causes you stress on an everyday basis, whether it's certain people or common situations. Are there ways you can avoid these stressors? If not, how can you reduce their impact on you? Here are some tips:

Minimize interpersonal stress. Unfortunately, other people can cause us lots of stress, and it's useless to try to change other people. With some people, you might want to minimize contact. With others, it's useful to try to understand why they act the way they do, and don't take their actions too personally. Even people whose company we enjoy can cause stress. Think carefully about how you want to spend your time and energy, and don't be afraid to say no to other people's requests for your time or energy.

Take a break. Make time for your hobbies. Take a stroll after dinner. Schedule a massage or aromatherapy session. Go to a concert. Take a scenic drive and turn the music on.

Take advantage of endorphins. Spend some time exercising. Hitting baseballs in a batting cage can be a great form of stress relief! Consider taking up the practice of yoga, pilates, tai chi, or some other form of relaxing movement. Virtually every health club, YMCA, and adult education program offers classes that teach such activities. Many hospitals do, as well.

Get your eight hours of sleep. When we're sleep deprived, we're likely to become stressed more easily. Fatigue can be a source of physical and emotional stress in its own right.

Relax your muscles. Tighten and release your muscles one group at a time, from face to toes, spending about ten seconds on each muscle group. This forces your muscles to relax. Simply knowing how your muscles feel when you are relaxed will make it easier for you to detect when you're feeling tense in response to stress.

CHAPTER 6
Your Drug Options

If you can't maintain good control with lifestyle tools alone, it's time to add medication to your arsenal. Your doctor can prescribe one or more medications that—when added to your ongoing diet and exercise regimen—can help. (Drugs for treating diabetes are used *in addition to*, not in place of, lifestyle changes.)

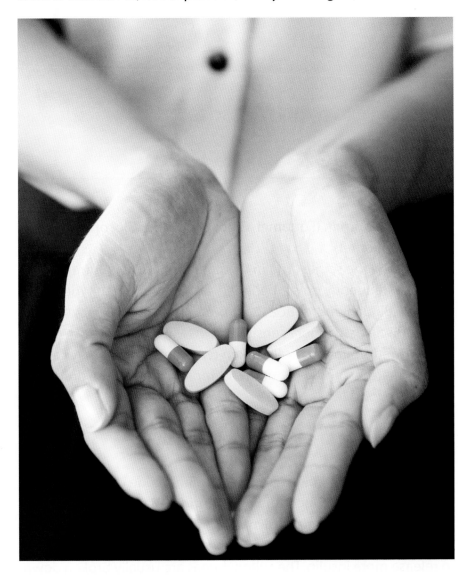

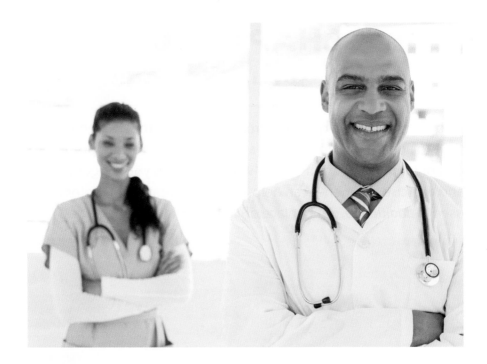

ORAL DRUGS

Biguanides

Includes: metformin (Fortamet, Glucophage and Glucophage XR, Glumetza, Riomet)

Metformin is the single drug in this category, and it is currently the most frequently prescribed medication for treating type 2 diabetes. Biguanides reduce sugar production in the liver and help make muscle tissue more sensitive to insulin so glucose can be absorbed. Metformin is typically taken two times a day. It may cause nausea, diarrhea, and gas, but this is improved when the drug is taken with food.

Sulfonylureas

Includes: chlorpropamide (Diabinese), glimepiride (Amaryl), glipizide (Glucotrol and Glucotrol XL), glyburide (Diabeta, Micronase) and micronized glyburide (Glynase)

Sulfonylureas work by stimulating the beta cells in the pancreas to release more insulin. The sulfonylureas are usually broken down into older "first generation" pills and newer "second generation" pills. First generation sulfonylureas have fallen out of favor because, in general, the second-generation versions are more potent and have fewer side effects. These medications are usually taken once or twice a day before meals. They will start working quickly to reduce your blood sugar, and they will not affect your blood pressure or cholesterol. Sulfonylureas have similar effects on blood glucose levels but differ in side effects, how often they are taken, and drug interactions.

Meglitinides
Includes: nateglinide (Starlix), repaglinide (Prandin)
Like sulfonylureas, meglitinides trigger the beta cells of the pancreas to release insulin. The difference is that meglitinides are impatient: They want that insulin released *now*. What's more, while sulfonylureas linger in the body all day, meglitinides rush in and out quickly. Because of their hyperactive nature, meglitinides play a specific role in managing type 2 diabetes: They are taken immediately before each of a day's three meals to boost insulin production in order to lower the predictable post-meal rise in blood sugar. Meglitinides appear to cause hypoglycemia less often than sulfonylureas do but hypoglycemia still a possibility, especially if the dose is too high. Meglitinides can also cause weight gain. Other side effects are uncommon but can include backaches, headaches, cold and flu symptoms, chest pain, gastrointestinal problems, joint pain, tingling skin, certain infections, and vomiting.

Thiazolidinediones (Glitazones or TZDs)
Includes: pioglitazone (Actos), rosiglitazone (Avandia)
This group of medications, sometimes referred to as insulin sensitizers, help insulin work better in the muscle and fat and also reduce glucose production in the liver. The Food and Drug Administration (FDA) ordered an early version of these drugs, called

troglitazone (under the brand name Rezulin), taken off the market in the United States in 2000 because it caused serious liver damage in rare cases. Rosiglitazone and pioglitazone have thus far not shown the same liver problems, although users are monitored closely as a precaution.

Alpha-Glucosidase Inhibitors (AGIs)
Includes: acarbose (Precose), miglitol (Glyset)
Alpha-glucosidase is a type of enzyme that lines the small intestine. Its job is to break down certain forms of sugar—starches, such as bread and potatoes, and sucrose, or table sugar—into glucose molecules small enough to pass into the bloodstream. Alpha-glucosidase inhibitors (AGIs) interfere with these enzymes, delaying the digestion and absorption of these sugars. These medications are taken with the first bite of food to help prevent post-meal sugar spikes. AGIs may have side effects, including flatulence, abdominal pain, and diarrhea.

DPP-4 Inhibitors
Includes: alogliptin (Nesina), linagliptin (Trajenta), saxagliptin (Onglyza), sitagliptan (Januvia)
This new class of oral diabetes medications helps to control blood sugar levels, particularly after meals. These drugs affect incretins, the hormones produced by the intestines that instruct the pancreas to make and release more insulin when you eat in order to keep the blood sugar levels from skyrocketing. One of the most important of these incretins is GLP-1. GLP-1 also aids blood sugar control by decreasing the amount of the hormone glucagon that the pancreas sends to the liver near mealtimes. Normally, an enzyme in the body called DPP-4 quickly turns off GLP-1 and the other incretins. The DPP-4 inhibitor medications block this enzyme, allowing GLP-1 to do a better job of keeping blood sugar levels in check.

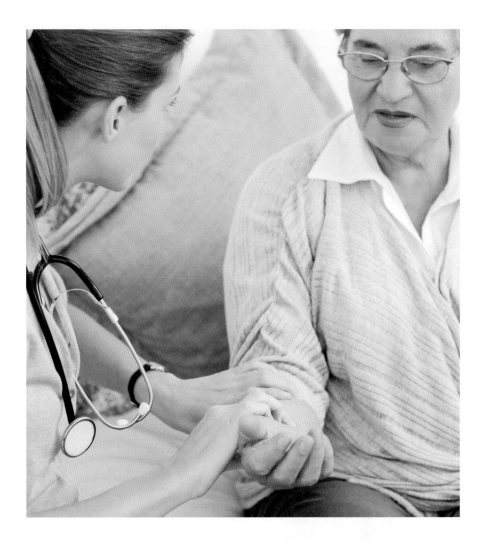

NON-INSULIN INJECTABLE DRUGS

Incretin Mimetics
Includes: exenatide (Byetta), Liraglutide (Victoza)
These medications stimulate insulin production while suppressing the liver's glucose output. They may decrease appetite and promote some weight loss. They can cause nausea, though it often fades over time. They usually do not cause hypoglycemia, though if you are taking a sulfonylurea, your doctor may reduce the dose of that to reduce the risk for hypoglycemia.

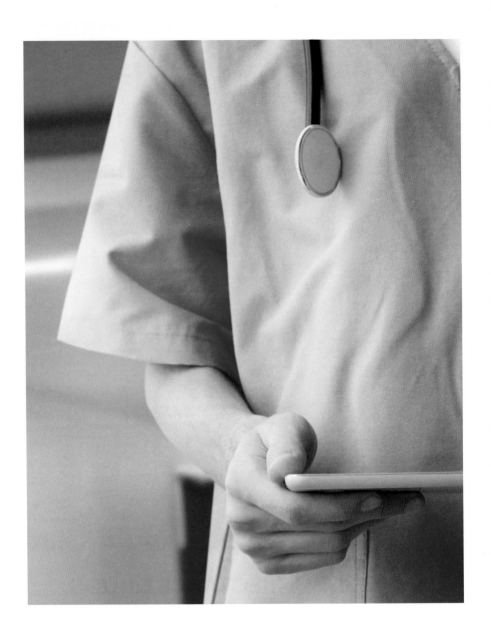

Amylin Mimetics

Includes: pramlintide (Symlin)

This medication slows digestion and helps prevent post-meal glucose spikes. Some users even lose a few pounds. It also reduces glucose production by the liver. It is injected before meals. The most common side effect is nausea, which usually reduces over time.

INSULIN THERAPY

When doctors abandoned the old name "non-insulin-dependent diabetes mellitus" in favor of the sleeker "type 2 diabetes," they weren't merely opting for a time-saving moniker. They were acknowledging that, for at least one-quarter of their patients with the condition, the old name is just plain wrong. Although most people with type 2 diabetes have a functioning pancreas when first diagnosed, over time their beta cells may not be able to keep up with demand for insulin, even if oral or noninsulin injectable diabetes drugs are added to diet and exercise therapy.

Research shows that oral medications are frequently not enough for patients to maintain healthy blood sugar. For instance, a 1998 British study of nearly 600 people with type 2 diabetes found that within three years of starting on metformin and a sulfonylurea, just one-third of patients had A1c readings below 7 percent. This is critical, as over the long term, levels higher than 7 percent can lead to organ damage. On the other hand, properly executed insulin therapy is just about foolproof, with a stellar track record for lowering blood sugar.

When blood tests reveal glucose levels that remain stubbornly high, doctors will usually advise insulin therapy. Although many physicians once considered insulin injections to be the treatment of last resort for their patients with type 2 diabetes, many now see this form of hormone replacement therapy as a way to better manage the disease at earlier stages in order to prevent the serious, debilitating complications that can result from chronically elevated blood sugar.

APPENDIX A
Carb Exchange List

1 vegetable exchange
(5 grams carbohydrate) equals:

½ cup	Vegetables, cooked (carrots, broccoli, zucchini, cabbage, etc.)
1 cup	Vegetables, raw, or salad greens
½ cup	Vegetable juice

1 milk exchange
(12 grams carbohydrate) equals:

1 cup	Milk: fat-free, 1% fat, 2%, or whole
¾ cup	Yogurt, plain nonfat or low-fat
1 cup	Yogurt, artificially sweetened

1 fruit exchange
(15 grams carbohydrate) equals:

1 small	Apple, banana, orange, or nectarine
1 medium	Peach
1 whole	Kiwi
½	Grapefruit or mango
1 cup	Berries, fresh (strawberries, raspberries, blueberries)
1 cup	Melon, fresh, cubes
1 slice	Melon, honeydew or cantaloupe
½ cup	Juice (orange, apple, or grape)
4 teaspoons	Jelly or jam

1 starch exchange
(15 grams carbohydrate) equals:

1 slice	Bread (white, pumpernickel, wholewheat, rye)
2 slices	Bread, reduced-calorie or "lite"
¼ (1 oz)	Bagel, bakery-style
½	Bagel, frozen, or English muffin
½	Bun, hamburger or hot dog
1 small	Dinner roll
¾ cup	Cold cereal
⅓ cup	Rice (cooked), brown or white
⅓ cup	Barley or couscous, cooked
⅓ cup	Legumes (dried beans, peas, lentils)
½ cup	Beans, cooked (black or kidney beans, chick peas)
½ cup	Pasta, cooked
½ cup	Corn, potato, or green peas
3 ounces	Potato, baked, sweet or white
¾ ounce	Pretzels
3 cups	Popcorn, air-popped or microwaved

1 meat exchange

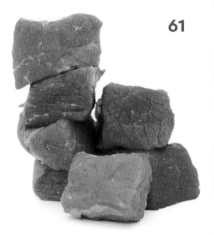

(0 grams carbohydrate) equals:

1 ounce	Beef, pork, turkey, or chicken
1 ounce	Fish fillet (flounder, sole, scrod, cod, etc.)
1 ounce	Tuna or sardines, canned
1 ounce	Shellfish (clams, lobster, scallops, shrimp)
¾ cup	Cottage cheese, nonfat or low-fat
1 ounce	Cheese, shredded or sliced
1 ounce	Lunch meat
1 whole	Egg
¼ cup	Egg substitute
4 ounces	Tofu

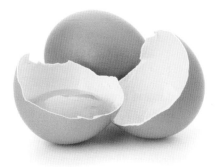

1 fat exchange

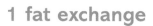

(0 grams carbohydrate) equals:

1 teaspoon	Oil (vegetable, corn, canola olive, etc.)
1 teaspoon	Butter
1 teaspoon	Margarine, stick
1 teaspoon	Mayonnaise
1 Tablespoon	Margarine or mayonnaise, reduced-fat
1 Tablespoon	Salad dressing
1 Tablespoon	Cream cheese
2 Tablespoons	Lite cream cheese
⅛	Avocado
8 large	Black olives
10 large	Green olives, stuffed
1 slice	Bacon

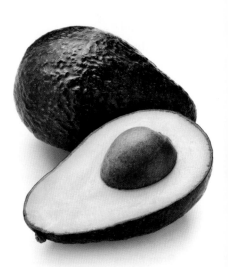

APPENDIX B Glycemic Index of Common Foods

Bread/Crackers

Bagel	72
Graham crackers	74
Hamburger bun	61
Kaiser roll	73
Pita bread	57
Pumpernickel bread	51
Rye bread, dark	76
Rye bread, light	55
Saltines	74
Sourdough bread	52
Wheat bread, high-fiber	68
White bread	71

Cakes/Cookies/Muffins

Angel food cake	67
Banana bread	47
Blueberry muffin	59
Chocolate cake	38
Corn muffin	102
Cupcake with icing	73
Donut	76
Oat bran muffin	60
Oatmeal cookie	55
Pound cake	54
Shortbread cookies	64

Candy

Jelly beans	80
Lifesavers	70
M&M's, peanut	33
Milky Way Bar	44

Cereals/Breakfast

All-Bran	42
Bran flakes	74
Cheerios	74
Cocoa Krispies	77
Corn flakes	83
Cream of wheat	70
Frosted Flakes	55
Golden Grahams	71
Grape Nuts	67
Life	66
Oatmeal	49
Pancakes	67
Puffed Wheat	67
Raisin Bran	73
Rice Bran	19
Rice Krispies	82
Shredded Wheat	69
Special K	66
Total	76
Waffles	76

Dairy

Chocolate milk	34
Ice cream, vanilla	62
Ice cream, chocolate	68
Milk, skim	32
Milk, whole	27
Soy milk	30
Yogurt, low-fat	33

Fruits/Juices

Apple	38
Apple juice	41
Apricot	57
Banana	55
Cantaloupe	65
Cherries	22
Cranberry juice	68